What to Expect When You're Expecting

by CONSTANCE BANNISTER

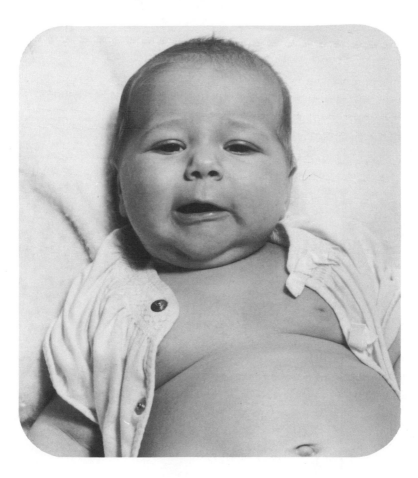

AN ESSANDESS SPECIAL EDITION
New York

What to Expect When You're Expecting

SBN-671-10299-0

What to Expect
When You're Expecting

by Constance Bannister

You're called "The Lady In Waiting,"
And your stomach doth protrude.
You waddle as you wait it out
And you crave the weirdest food.
You endure your stretch in silence;
You never would complain.
But your husband groans with the agonies
Of sympathetic pain.
The in-laws argue back and forth
What name your heir shall bear;
And your husband paces endlessly
While pulling out his hair.
Just disregard this side-line play
While the babies of Bannister fame
Amuse and entertain you
As you play this waiting game.

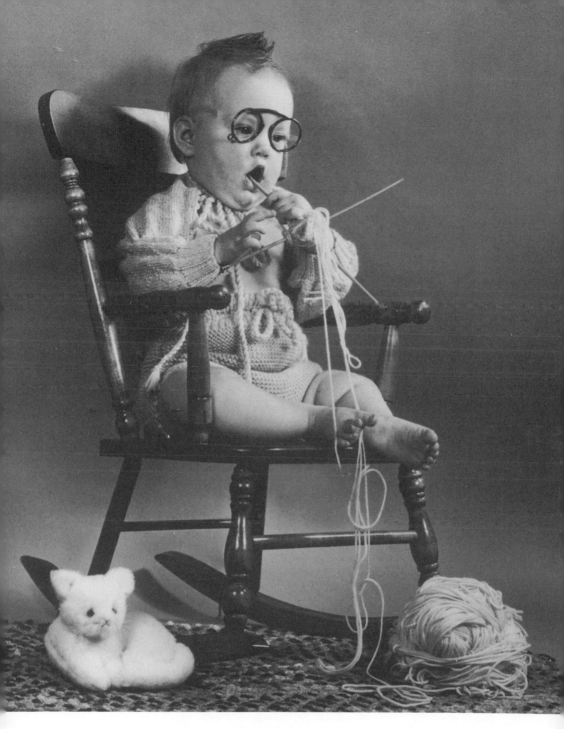

Come into the living room, dear;
I have something to tell you.

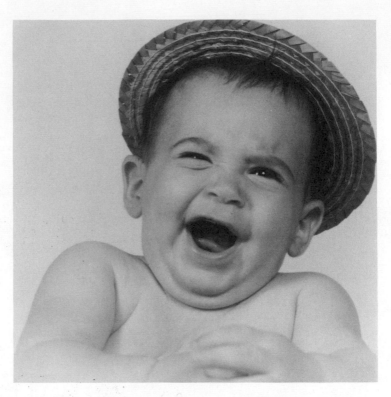

I'm happy, honey; I'm happy.
See, I'm laughing.

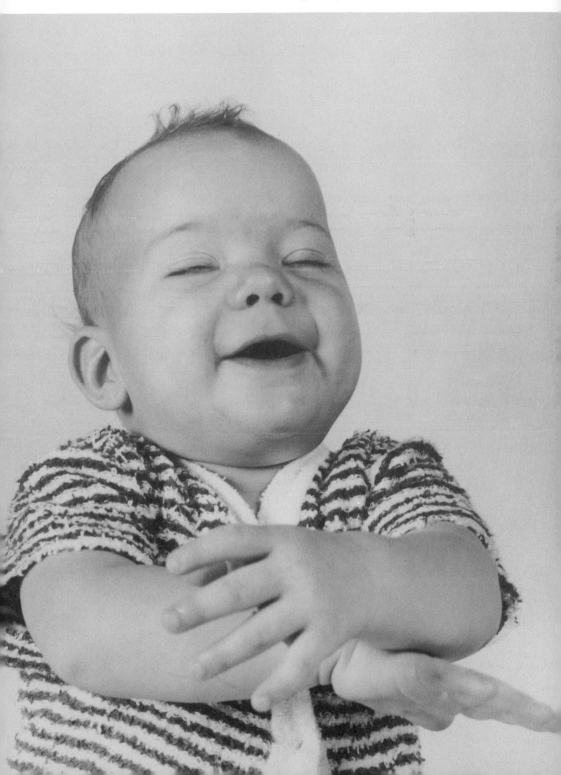

Wait 'til I tell the boys
down at the bowling alley.

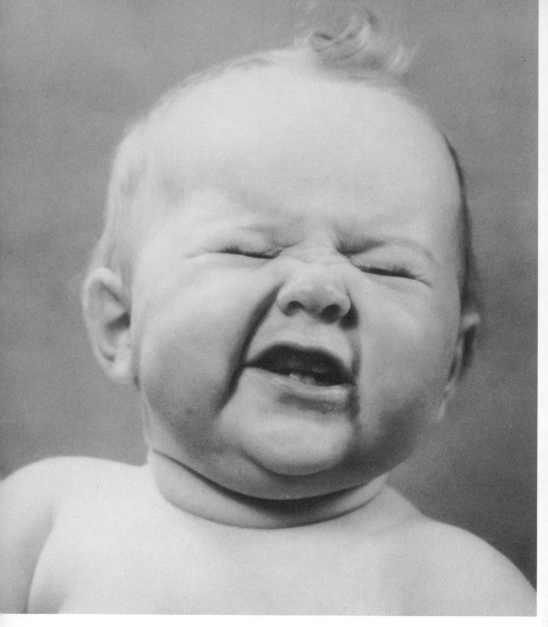

The medicine for <u>morning</u> sickness
is worse than the morning sickness.

The dame's going to drive me crazy
for the next seven months.

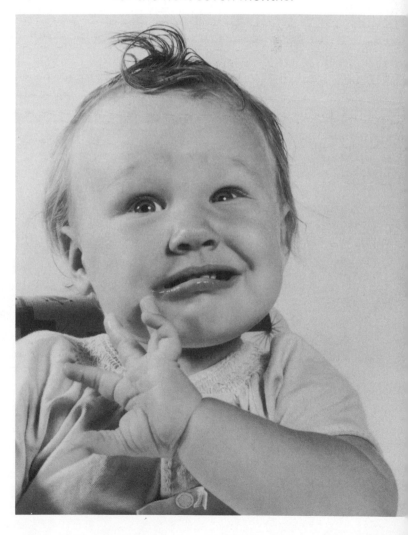

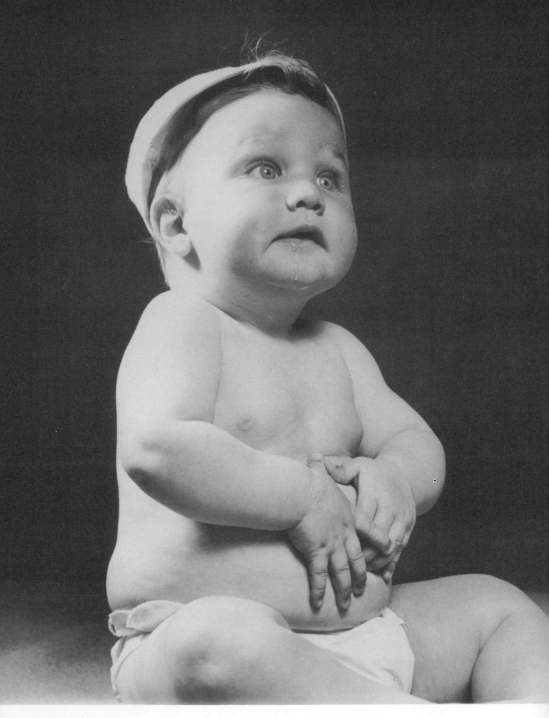

Call the office and tell them I won't be in today.
I've got morning sickness, too.

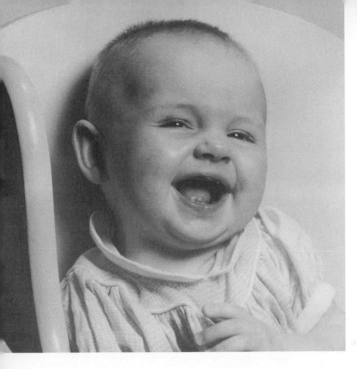

Mabel told me heartburn
is a sign the baby's hair
is growing.

This is my sixth popsicle today,
and I never liked ice cream before.

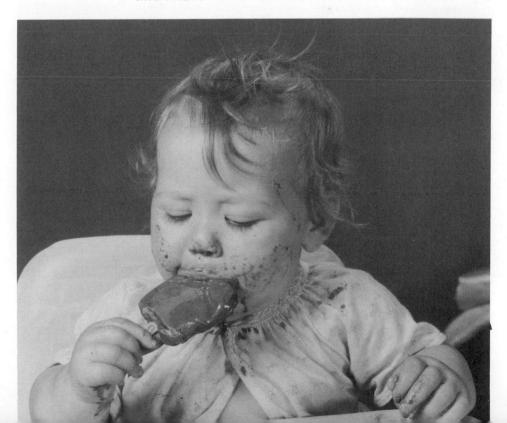

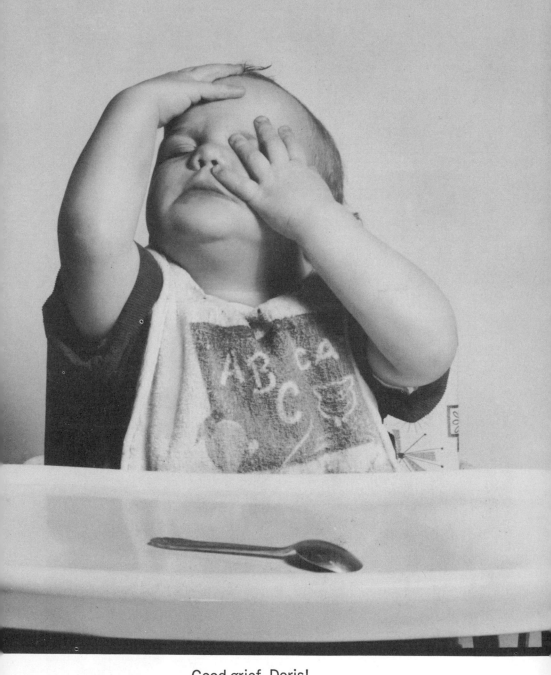

Good grief, Doris!
Please don't discuss your condition at dinner!

Aren't you going to wait on me hand and foot?
Remember, these first few months are difficult.

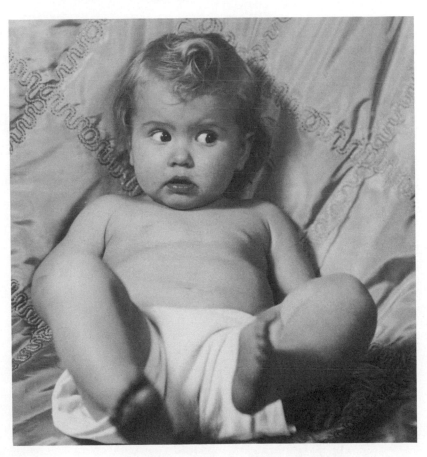

Don't wake me up just to tell me you're hungry.
You could scare a guy to death!

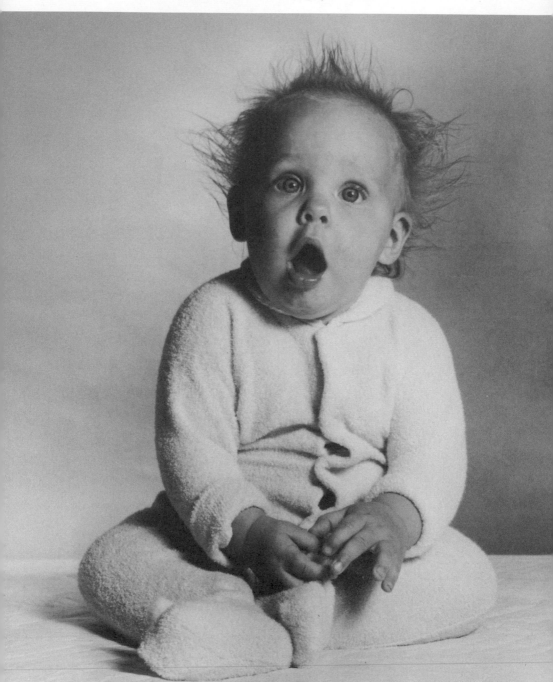

Do you think my figure's as good
as it was ten weeks ago?

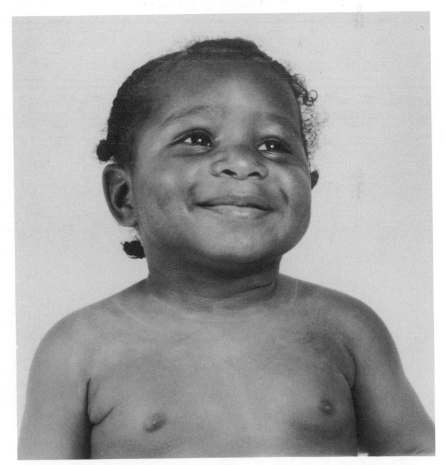

Jerry bet me a martini
you'd have a boy,
but I had to buy him
three martinis
before he'd bet.

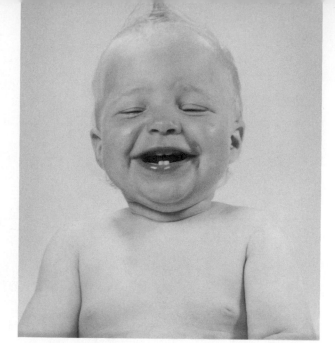

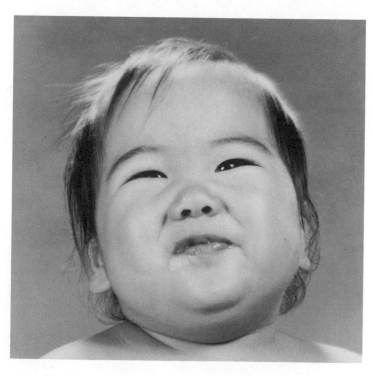

What's so remarkable about having a baby?
It's the same as it always was!

The Welcome Wagon is furnishing free diaper service
for a week!!

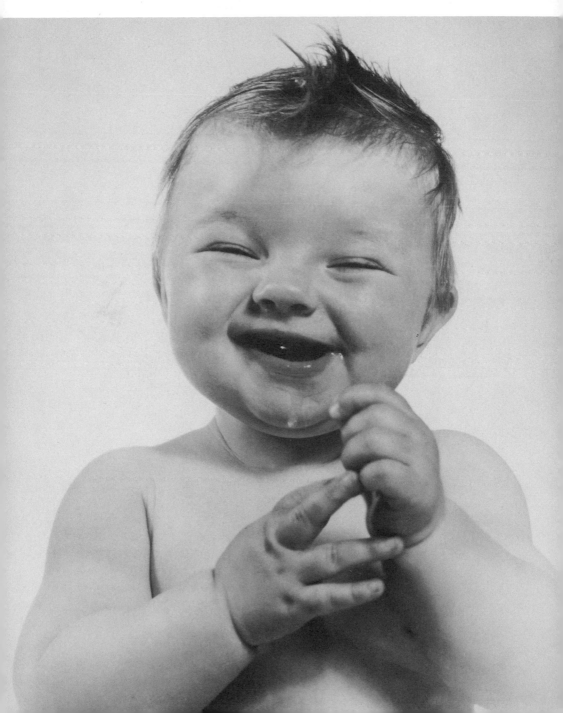

I <u>know</u> I cry easily.
First pregnancy is a traumatic experience.

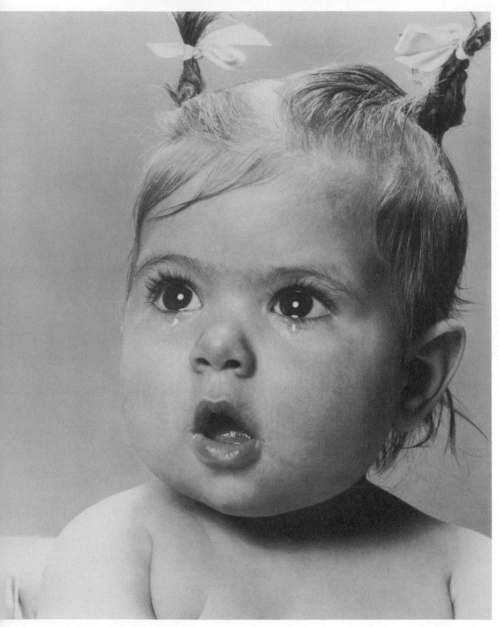

My fingers swelled so bad,
I can't get my wedding ring on.

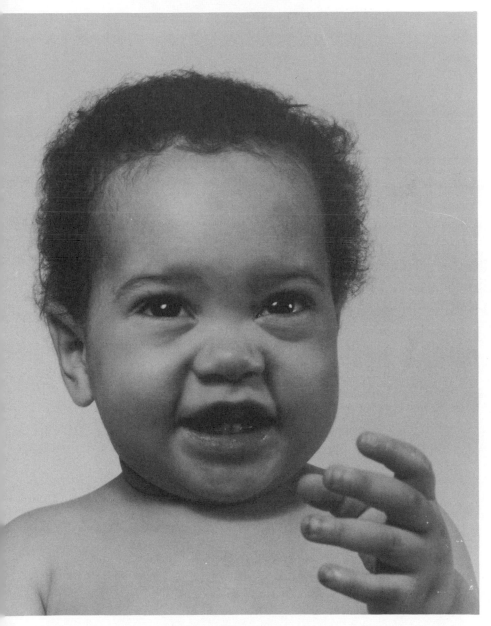

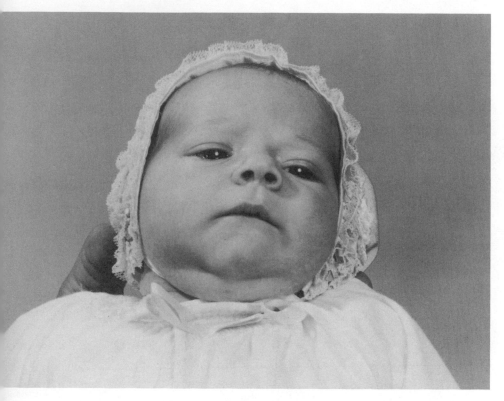

I'm only a mother-in-law.
Why should I know anything about having children?

Settle down, tiger,
and let's both get some sleep.

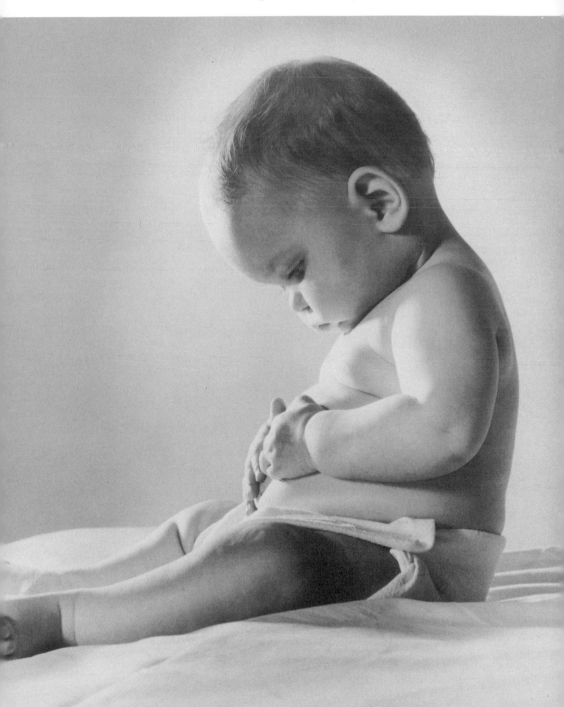

With all that kicking,
I'd say you're either going to have a ballerina
or an all-star quarterback!

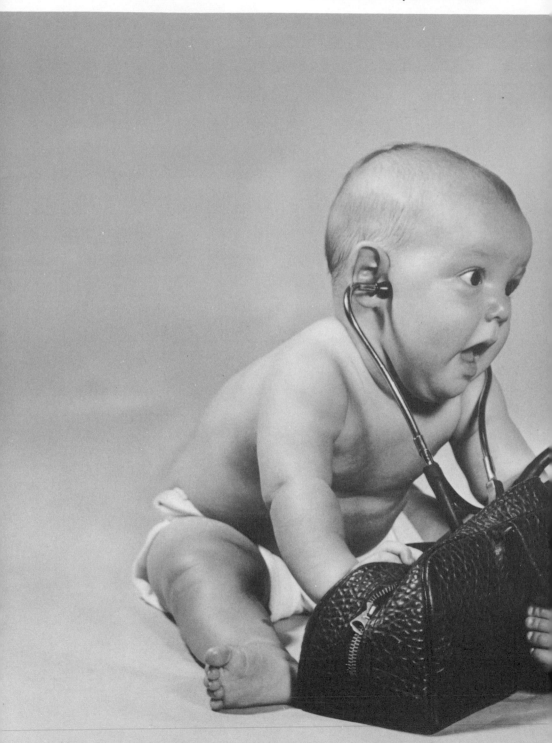

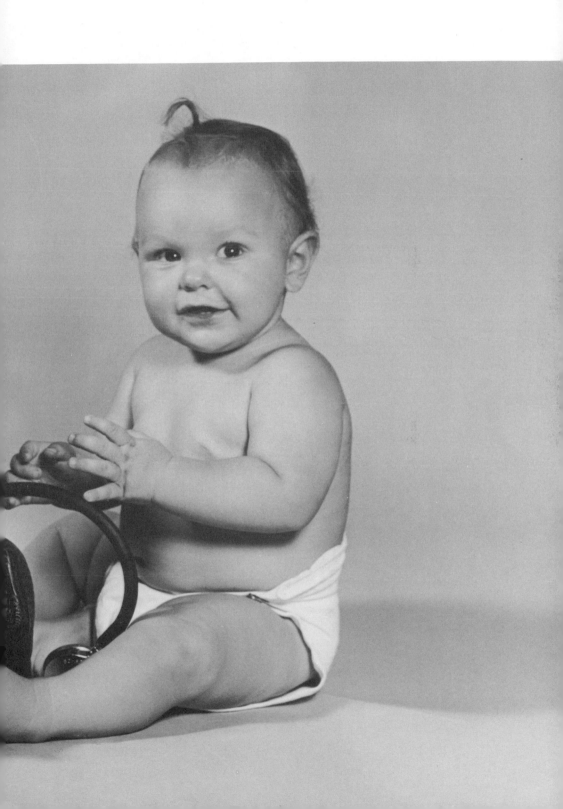

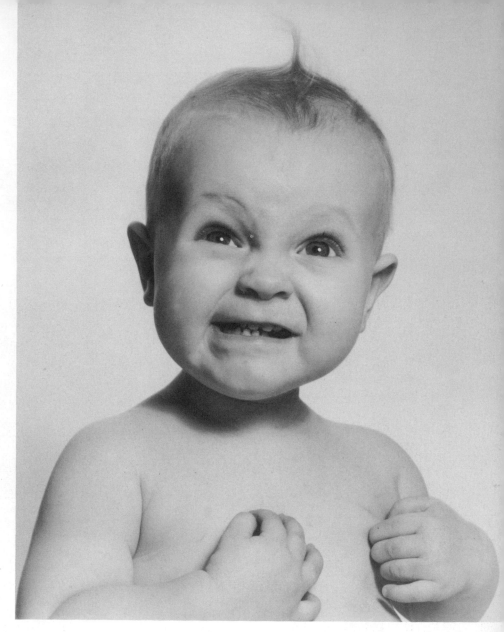

Won't nursing ruin my bustline, doctor?

I thought a new hat would be good for my morale
and would take the emphasis off the rest of me!

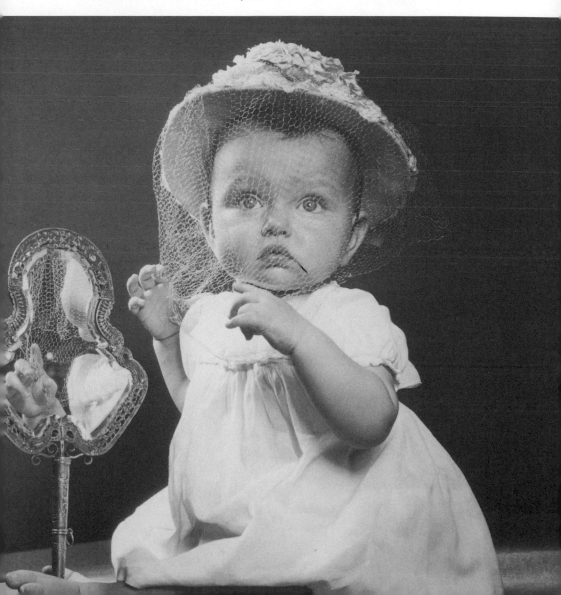

Let'see, we've got the crib,
the bathinette, sheets, diapers, bottles, etc., etc.
All we need now is the baby!

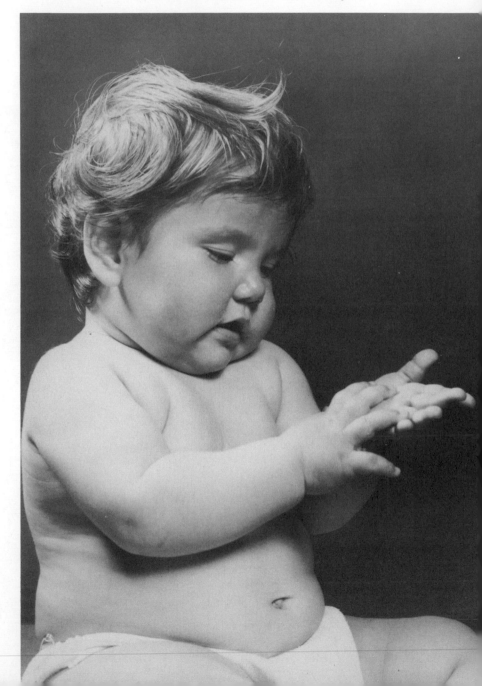

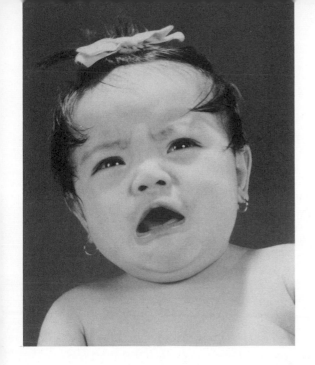

It's more than a month
since you've taken me out,
George. Are you ashamed
to be seen with me?

Suppose the guys
at the tavern
find out I'm going
to Expectant
Fathers School!

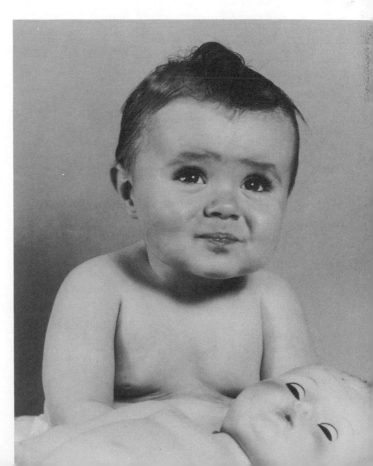

Your mother's moving in? Doesn't she think
I can handle the situation?

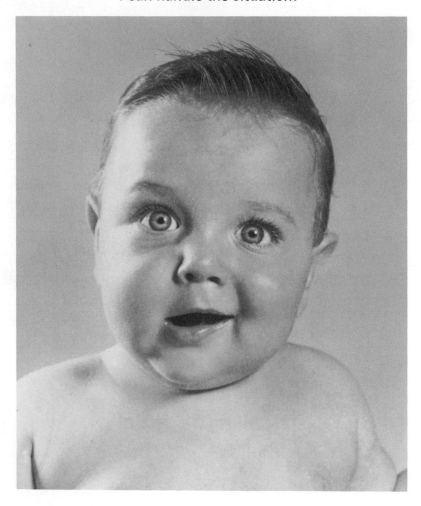

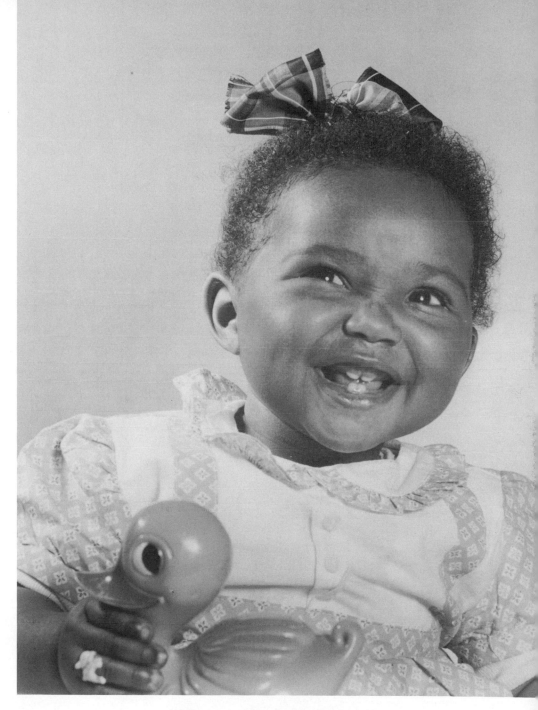

The nursery's so full of toys now,
there's no room for the baby!

Take it easy, my dear. The baby won't be here
for another eight weeks.

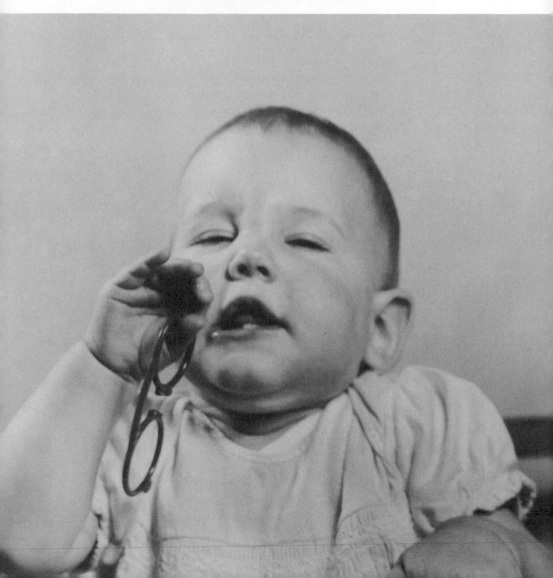

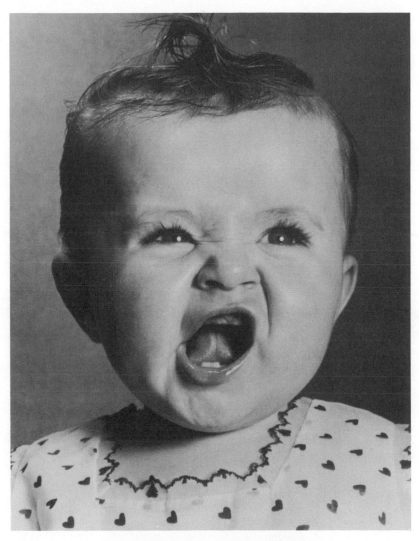

I don't care if he _is_ your doctor.
I'm your MOTHER,
and I know about babies, too!

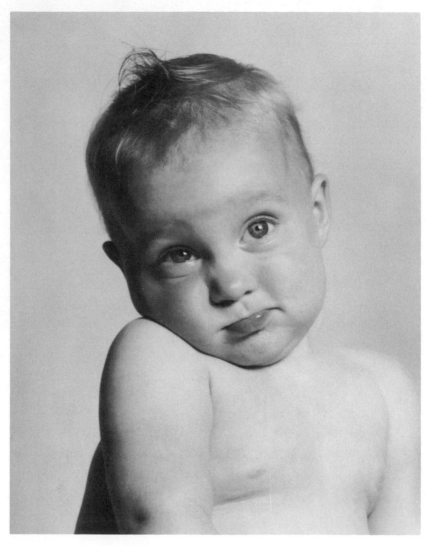

Couldn't we afford a nurse
just for the first two weeks?

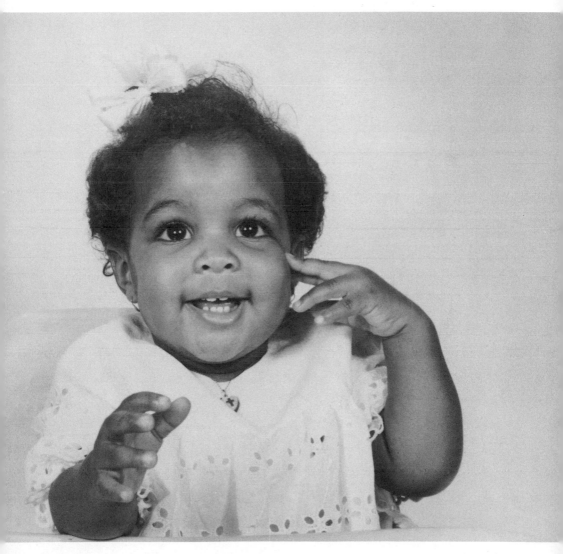

I've got the problem licked.
I'll paint the nursery walls blue,
and paint the furniture pink!

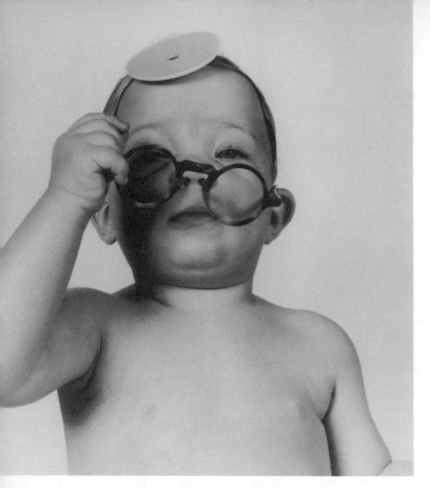

Everything about your pregnancy is normal except your desire to see the doctor so often!

You want pickled pigs' feet with whipped cream and chocolate sauce? I'm getting sick!

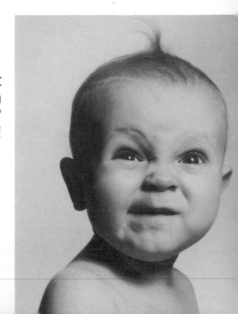

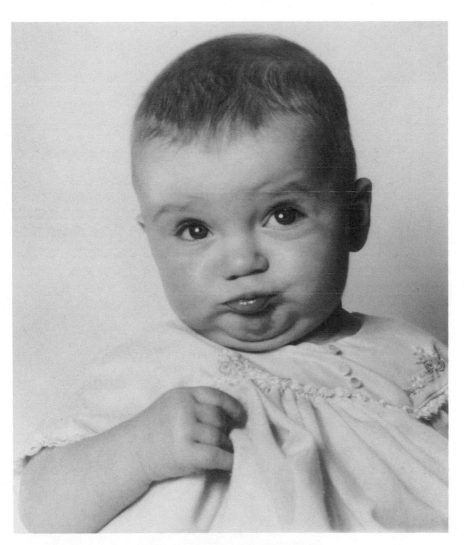

Even the maternity clothes
are starting to feel tight!

If I have a choice, God,
will you please make it a boy!!

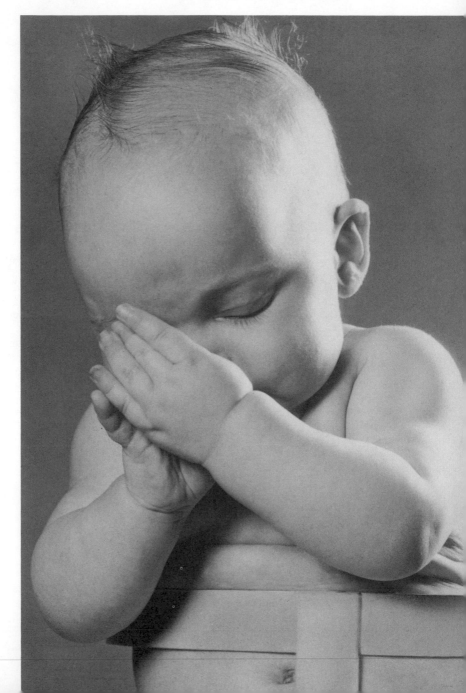

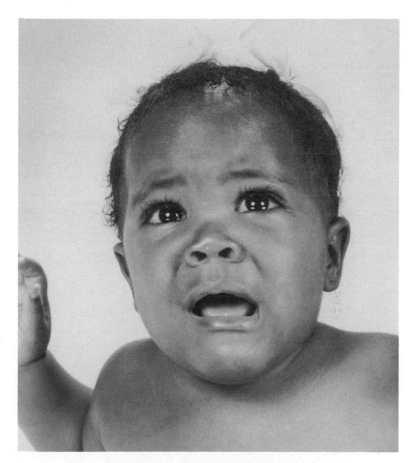

Tell me I look pregnant,
but <u>don't</u> tell me I look <u>fat</u>!!

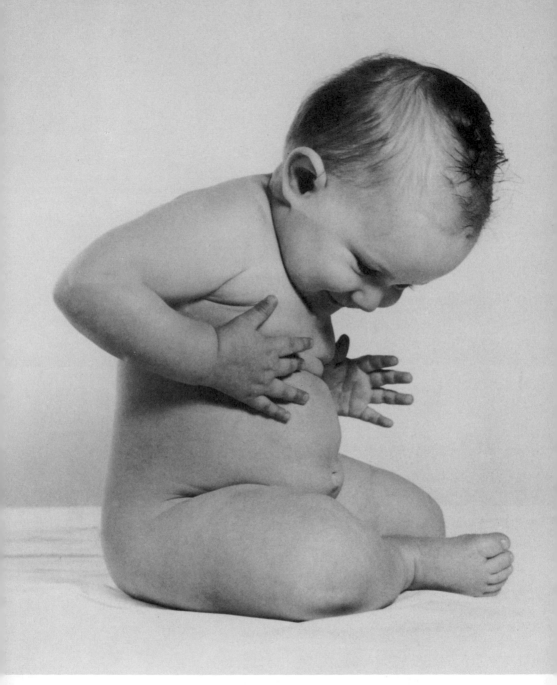

Sure it's water,
but there's a little fish
swimming in it!

I washed everything
in the nursery again today!

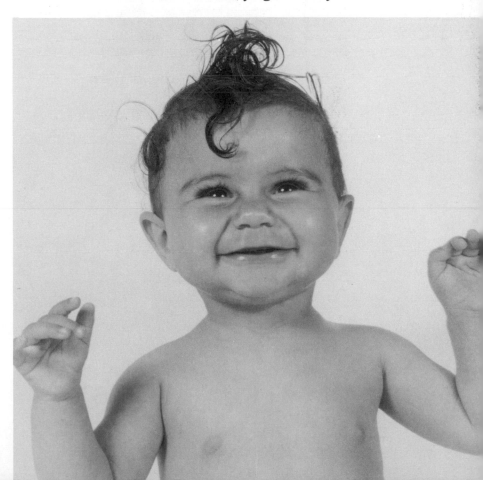

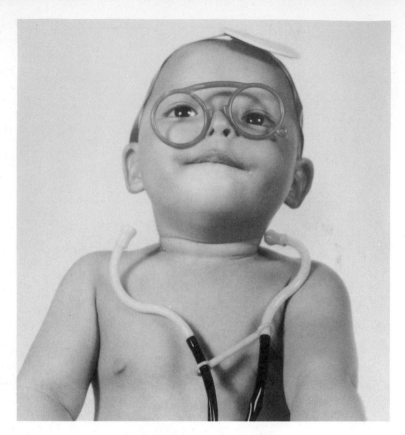

I'd say the little bundle
will arrive right on target.

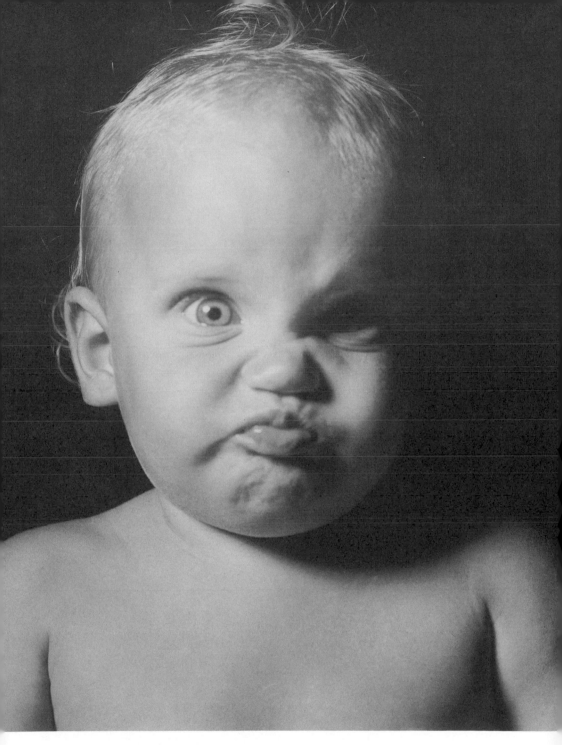

You don't need another maternity dress.
The baby will be here in another few weeks.

I got a check from my father
to cover all the extra expenses.

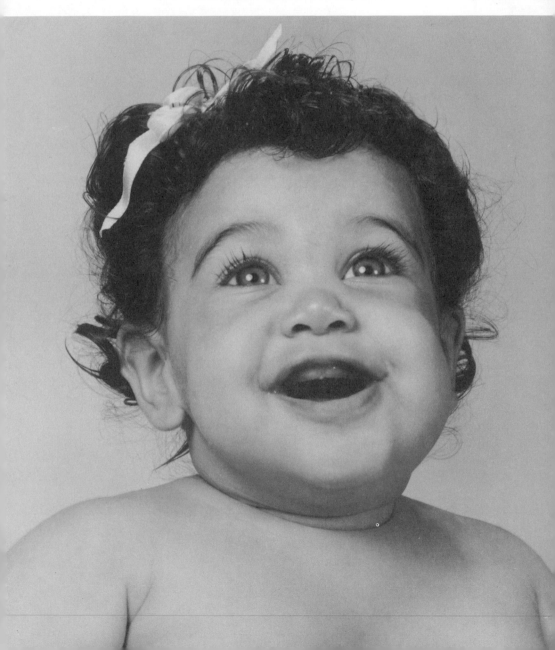

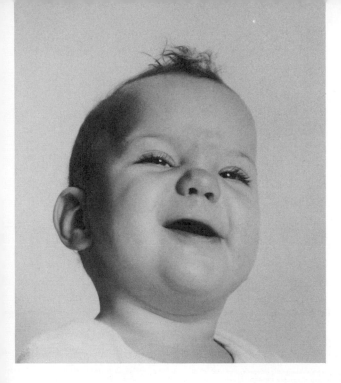

I don't mean
to hurt your feelings,
Alice,
but you're walking
just like a duck!

Two more weeks,
doctor?
It feels like
it's been two years
already!!

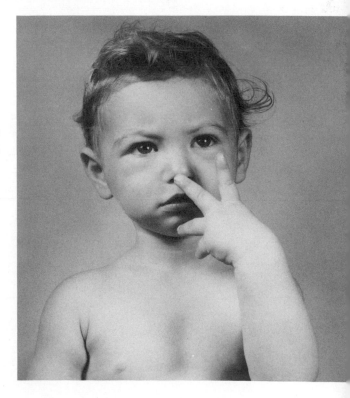

Honey, I just had another pain.
Please stay close to me now!

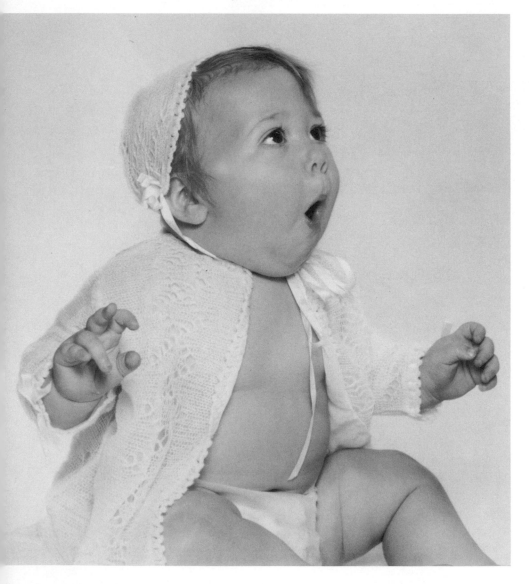

Seems like my fat stomach
has been pushing us apart!

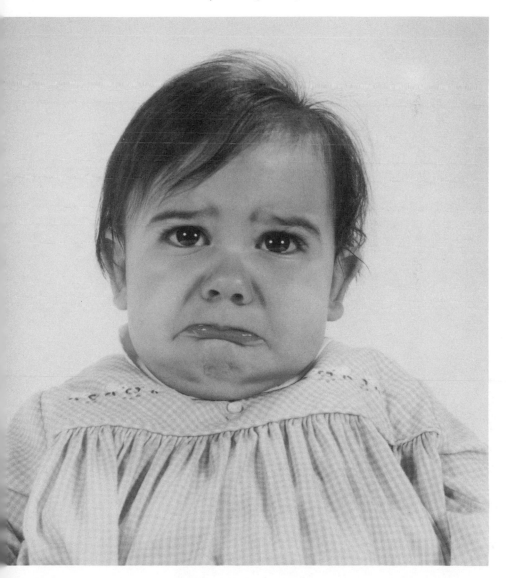

Who do you think watered your plants
when you had your tonsils out?

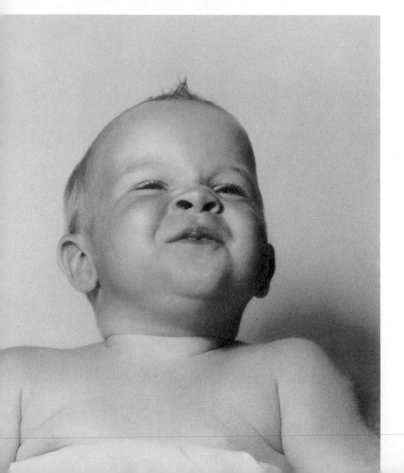

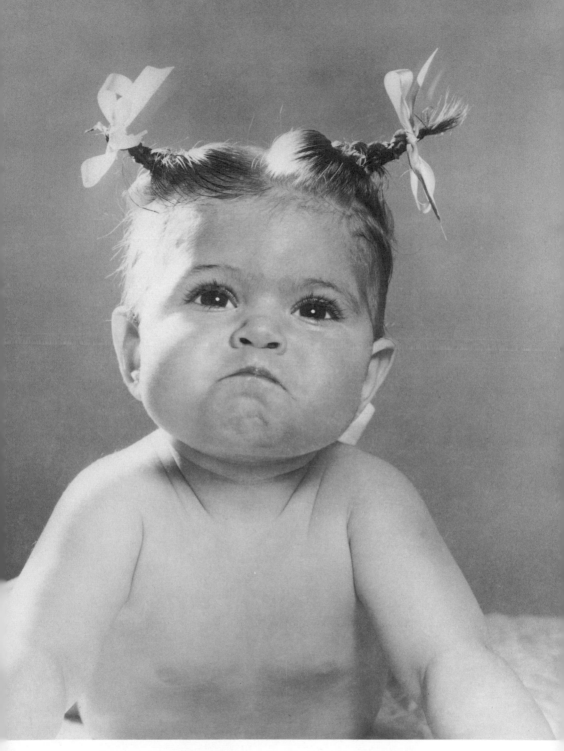

You are <u>not</u> going on a business trip, Charley.
The baby could come at any moment.

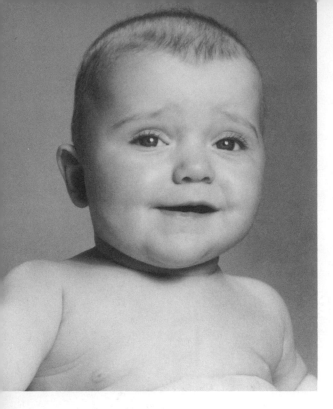

I'll use
the old squeeze play—
put the baby nurse
in the guest room
and my mother-in-law
can't stay over!

I don't care if
that <u>is</u> your father's name—
Marion sounds
like a girl to me!

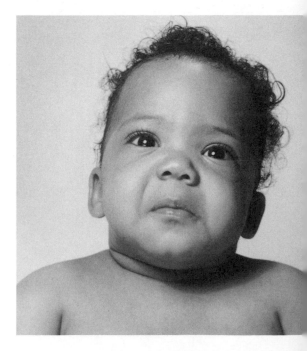

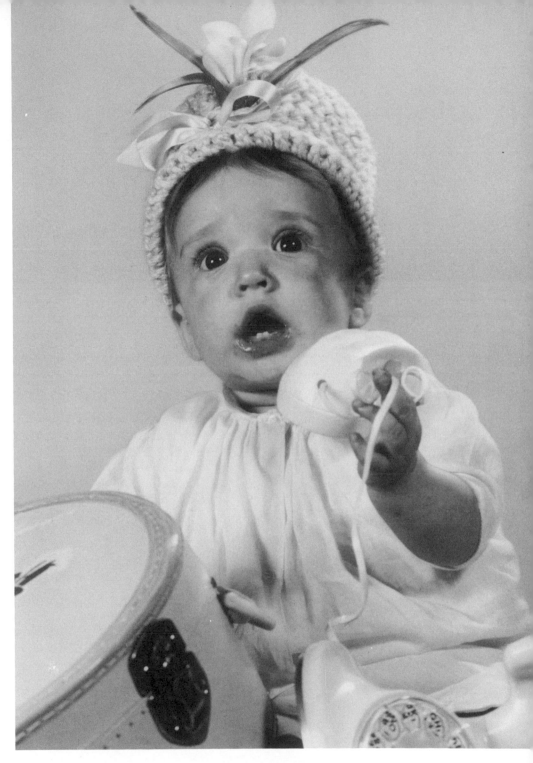

I have a feeling
there isn't time to repack!!

I think I'll just doze in the chair
'til you tell me you're ready to go.

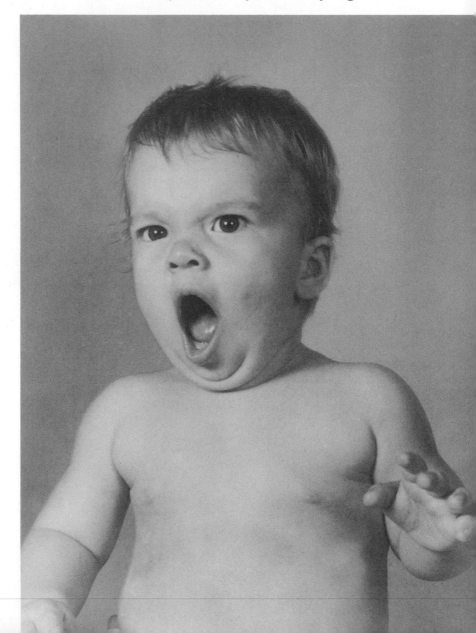

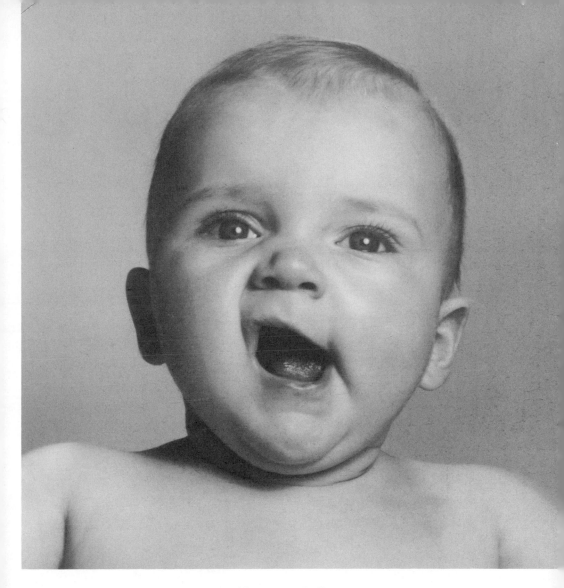

Hang on, lady.
This taxi ain't a maternity ward!!

I'll just whip over to the hospital and have the baby.
He's too nervous to drive anyway.

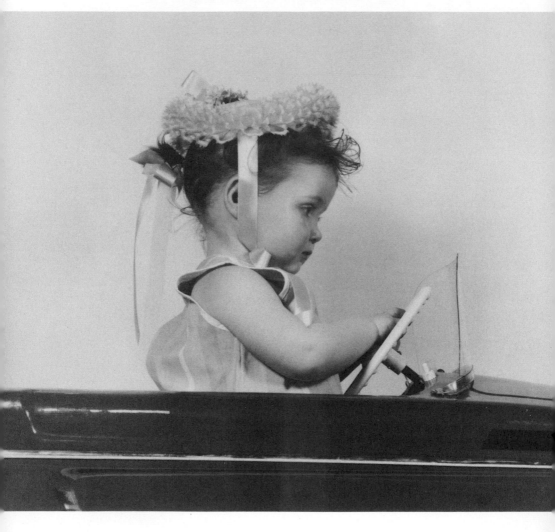

I feel like
a vine-ripened watermelon.

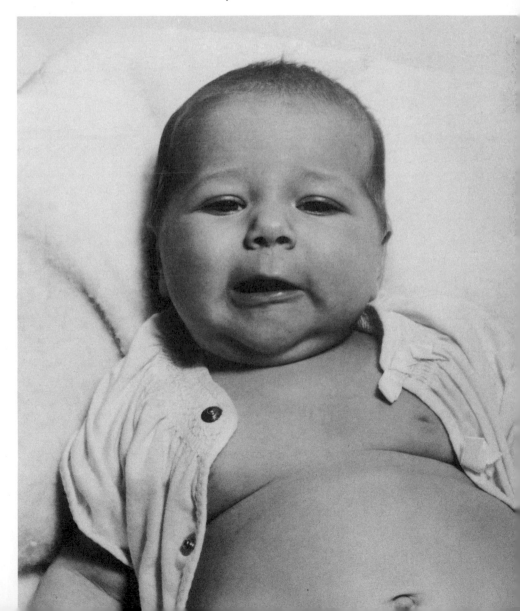

How long have <u>you</u> been in labor?

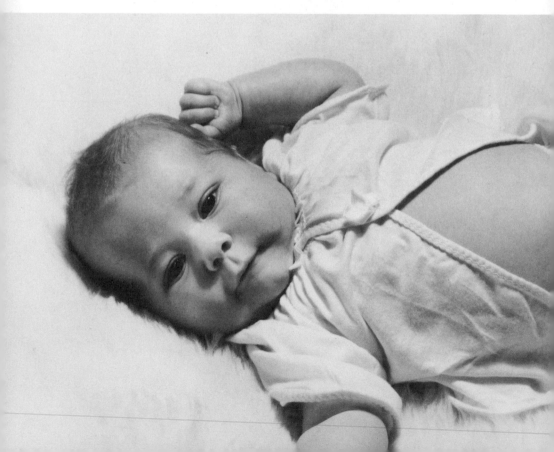

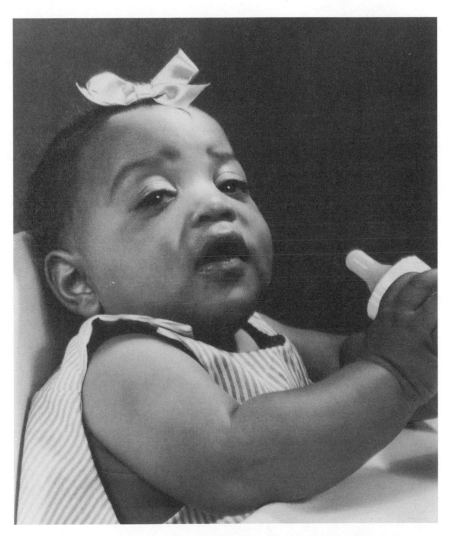

Who needs tranquilizers? If I were any more relaxed
I'd fall apart!

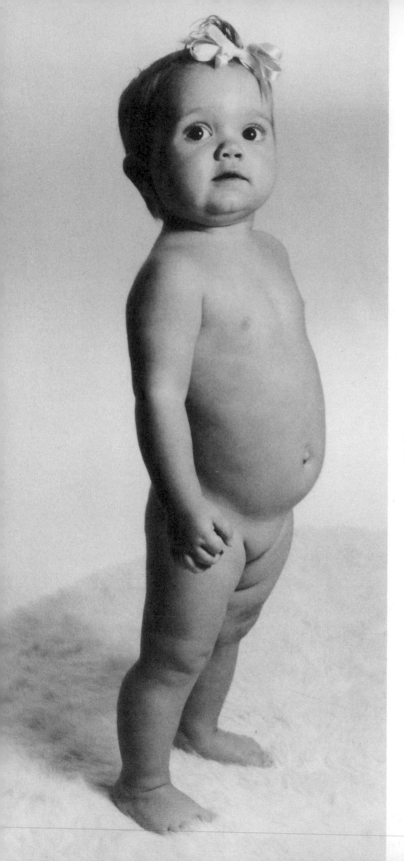

You'll have
no trouble
getting back
your figure.
Look at me,
and I've had
eight kids!

Guess what!
My canasta club is giving you
a baby shower!

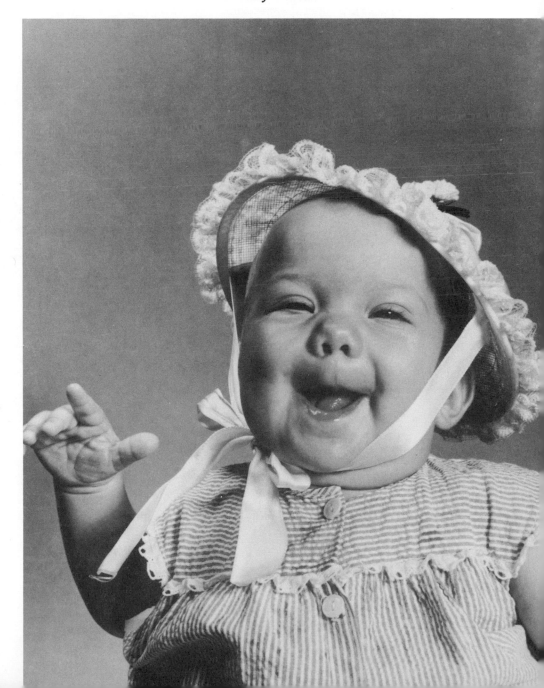

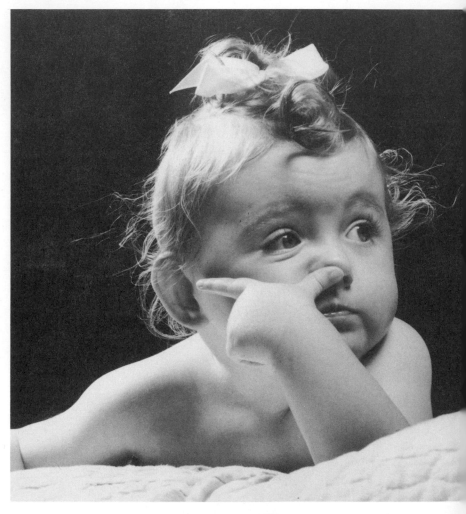

I might as well enjoy
these few days of rest.
It's the last I'm going to have
for a long time!

Five hours of pacing
and three packs of cigarettes.
I feel sick!

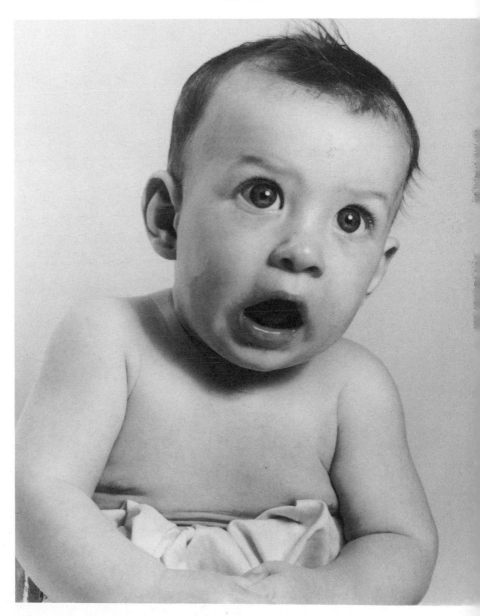

With your cast-iron constitution,
Mrs. Frobisher,
natural birth should be a snap!

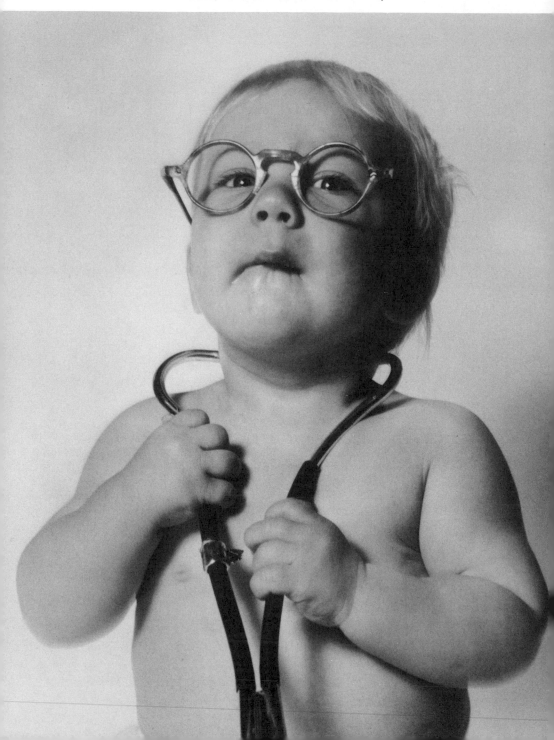

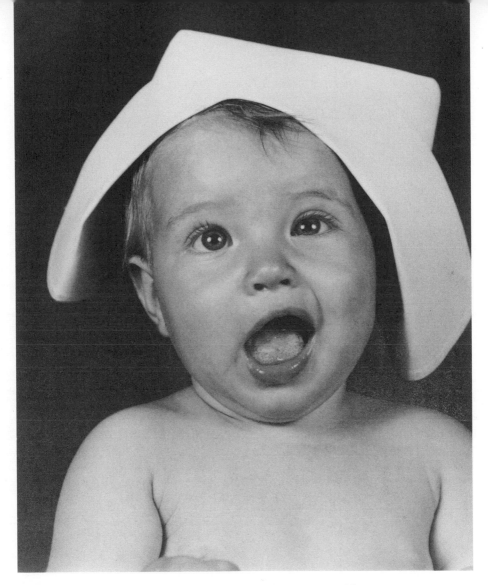

The least you could do is try…!!!

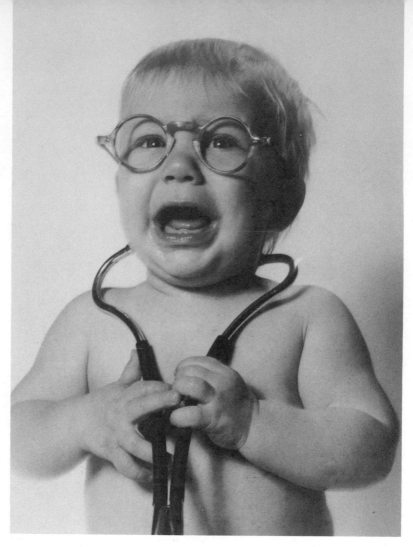

Why do all my patients sign in
at the same time?

Are cigars in order
if it's a girl?

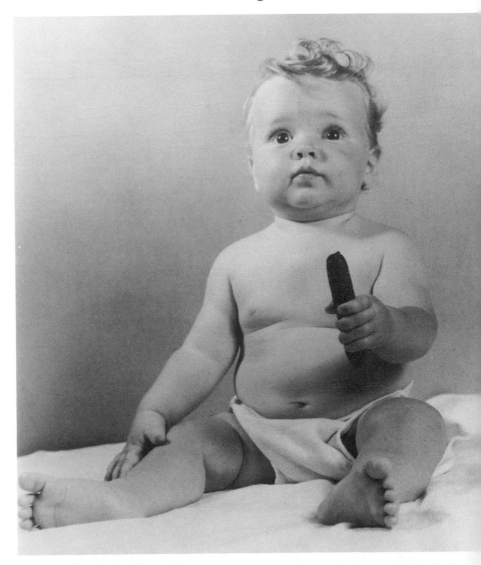

No, no, Mr. Wilson,
not five minutes. Five <u>children</u>—
you're the father of quintuplets!

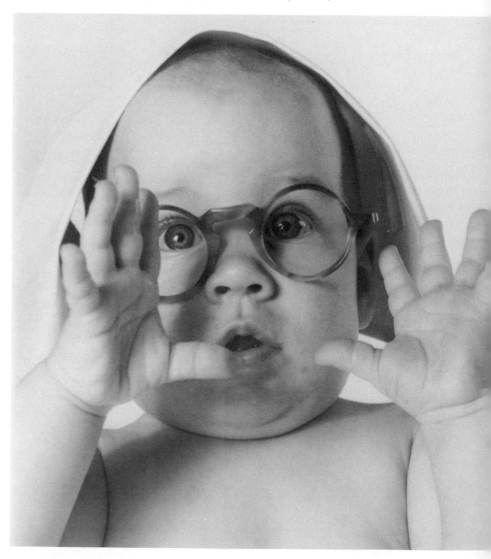

There isn't a baby
in this hospital that can hold
a candle to him!

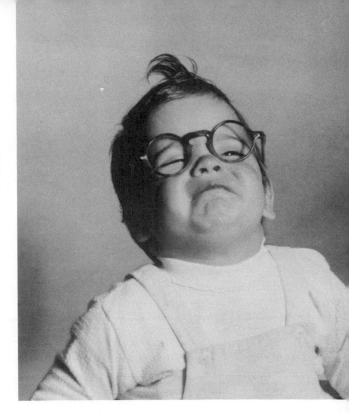

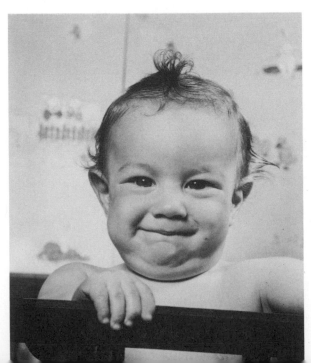

You look just like
your old man,
you good lookin' kid!!

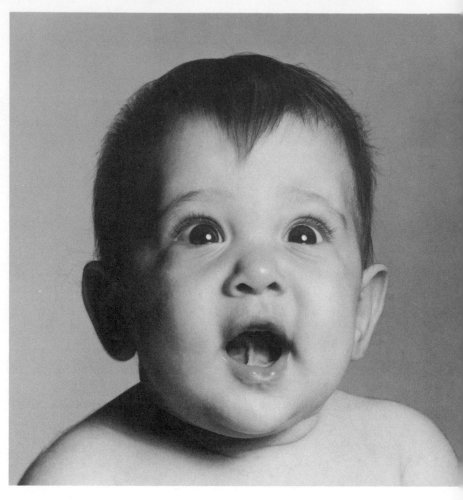

How many years do I have to wait
to discuss something beside the baby?

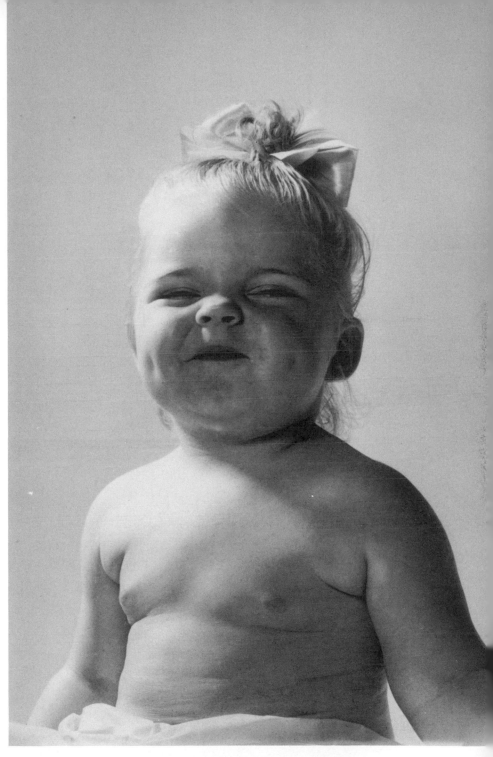

After the baby gets used to us,
you and I
are going to get used to each other again.

Oh, it's so good
to have you home again, dear!

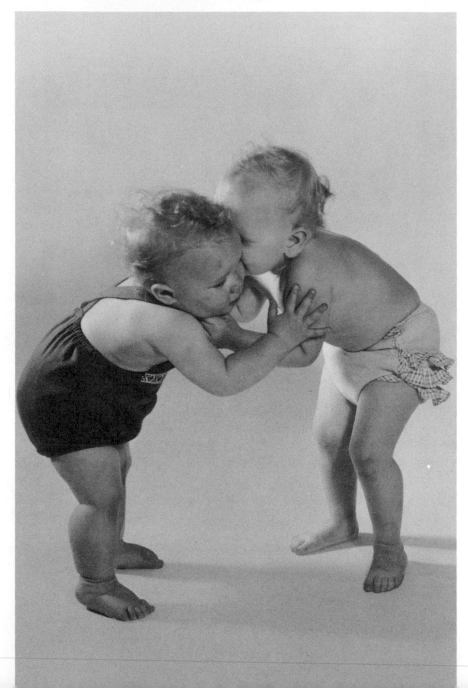

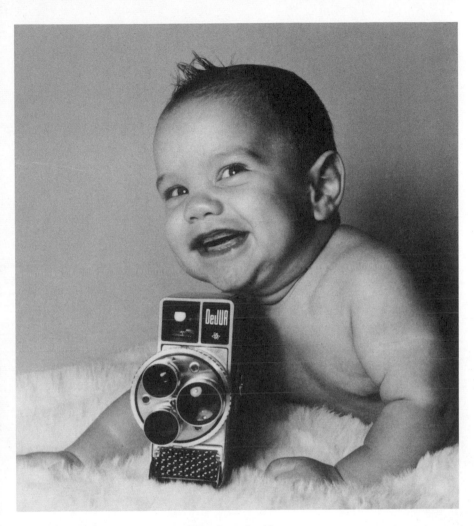

What a shot!
This kid of ours could be
a cover girl!

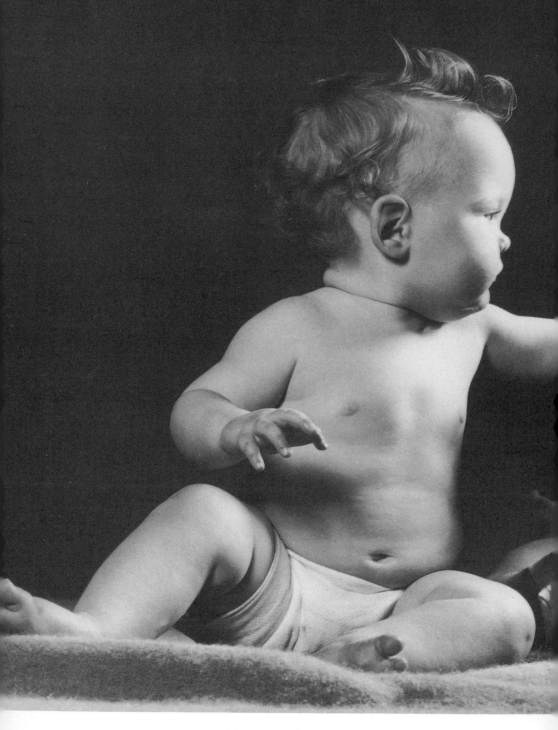

Honey, wake up!
It's your turn for
the four o'clock feeding!

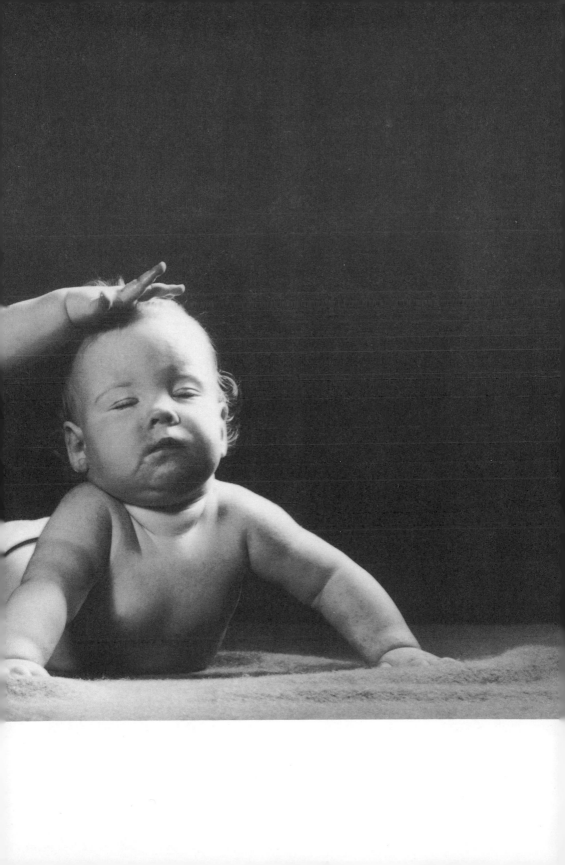

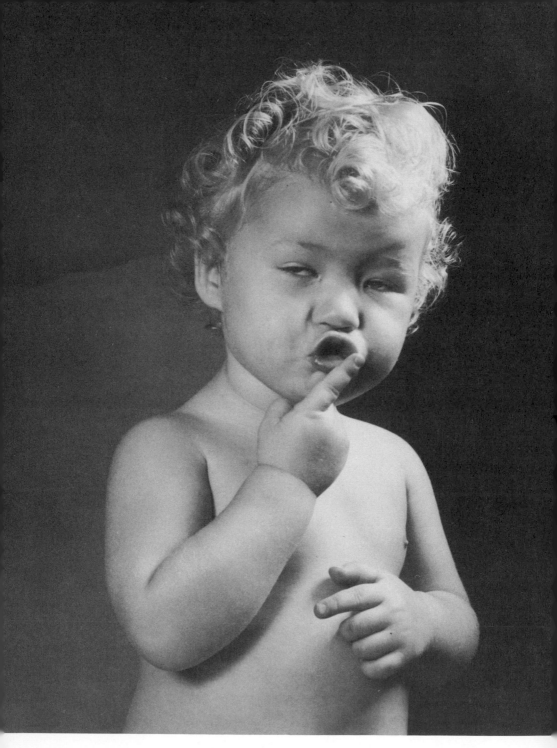

Shush!!
I finally got the baby to sleep!

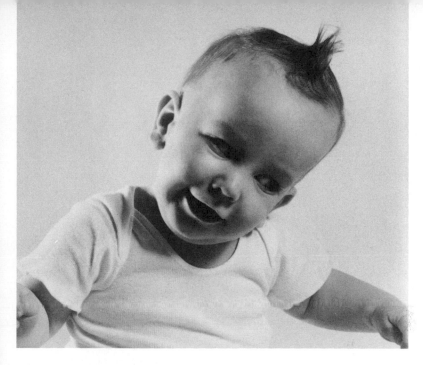

Will you
tell daddy
someday
where you
got red,
curly hair?

Four months of push-ups
and knee-bends and I've still got a pouch
like a mama kangaroo!

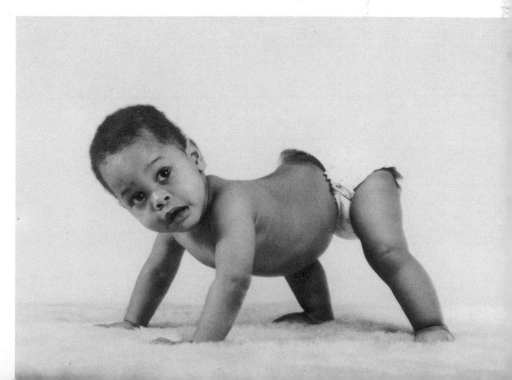

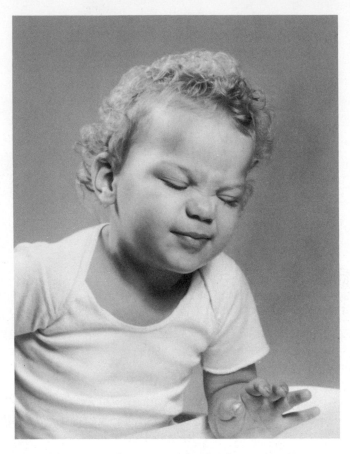

How could anyone who looks so sweet
smell so bad?

Here, devoted father.
<u>You</u> change her!

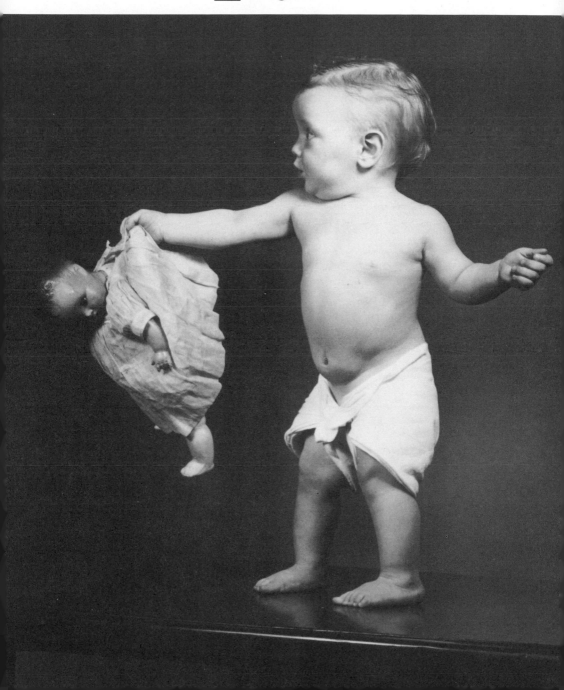

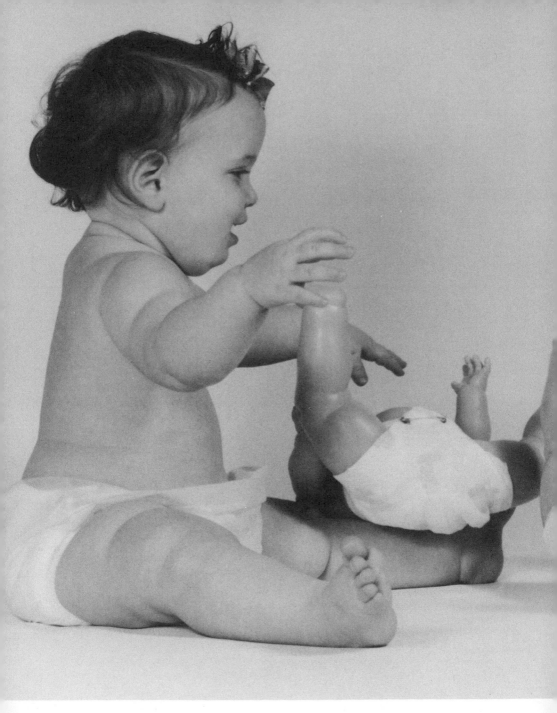

Are you two guys having a contest
to see which one drives Mother
up the wall?

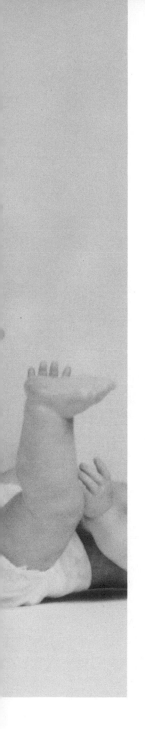

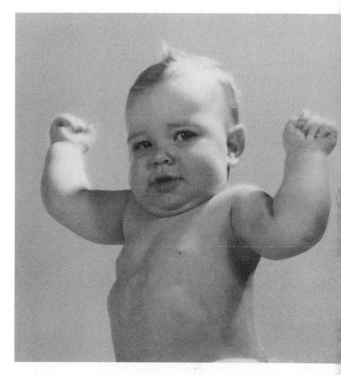

He's only three months old,
and he's got muscles as big as mine!

If I don't get a night's sleep soon,
I'm going to send myself a telegram and call myself
out of town on business!

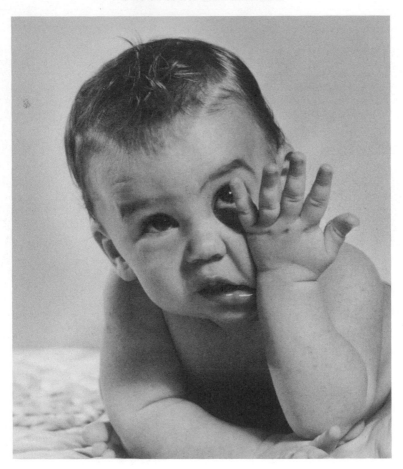

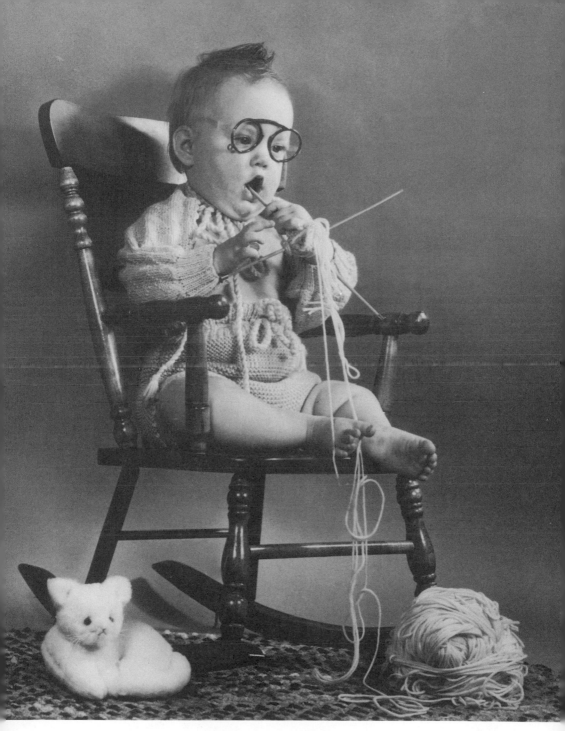

I might as well tell him
the same way I did the first time...

The shock won't be so great.

Here are six hilarious picture books by America's leading baby photographer, Constance Bannister, bringing you an irresistible collection of infant infamy bound to delight anyone this side of the playpen.

Bring on the laughter by buying one or all of these books. Purchase them from your favorite bookseller or fill in the coupon below and send it with your check to Simon & Schuster, Inc., Dept. CB-2, 11 West 39th Street, New York, N.Y. 10018. Do it today, now! (On orders of 3 or more books, do not include postage and handling charges.)

A diet book ▶ to end all diet books

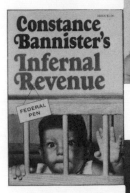

◀ zany fun for taxpayers

a rib-tickling ▶ topical satire

◀ a wild, wacky spoof of hospital life

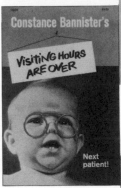

office ▶ politics unmasked

◀ a most engaging engagement book

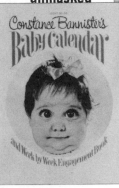
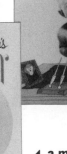

To your bookseller, or
Simon & Schuster, Inc., Dept. CB-2
11 West 39th Street, New York, N.Y. 10018

I enclose $_____ for

No. of
copies

_____ **IT'S A RIOT TO DIET, $1.00,** #10087

_____ **FROM THE BACK OF THE INCUBATOR, $1.00,** #10113

_____ **THE ORGANIZATION BABY, $1.00,** #10191

_____ **VISITING HOURS ARE OVER, $1.00,** #10235

_____ **INFERNAL REVENUE, $1.00,** #10264

_____ **BABY CALENDAR AND WEEK BY WEEK ENGAGEMENT BOOK, $2.00,** #10297

plus $.15 postage and handling charges on orders of 2 or less. (Residents of New York, New Jersey, and Illinois, please add applicable sales tax.)

Please send the books to

Name_____
                    (please print)

Address _____

City_____State_____Zip Code_____